RENAL DIET COOKBOOK FOR STAGE 4

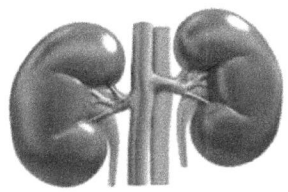

Effortless and Tasty Recipes with Low Potassium, Phosphorus, and Sodium, plus Food Lists and Meal Plans to Manage Kidney Disease

Fortune Flourish

Copyright © 2024 by Fortune flourish

All rights reserved. No part of this book may be reproduced, stored in a retrieval system, or transmitted in any form or by any means—electronic, mechanical, photocopying, recording, scanning, or otherwise—without the prior written permission of the publisher, except for brief quotations embodied in critical reviews and certain other noncommercial uses permitted by copyright law.

TABLE OF CONTENT

Introduction 5

    Understanding Stage 4 kidney disease 5

CHAPTER ONE 10

    Overview of Kidney Function 10

    Stages of Chronic Kidney Disease (CKD............. 11

CHAPTER TWO 17

    Nutritional Guidelines for Stage 4 kidney disease
    17

CHAPTER THREE 23

    Getting Started 23

    Meal Planning Tips 25

CHAPTER FOUR 29

    Breakfast Recipes 29

CHAPTER FIVE 37

    Lunch Recipes... 37

CHAPTER SIX.. 46

Dinner Recipes 46

CHAPTER SEVEN 55

Snack and Side Dish Recipes 55

CHAPTER EIGHT 61

Dessert Recipes 61

CHAPTER NINE 68

Beverages 68

CHAPTER TEN 75

SPECIAL OCCASIONS AND HOLIDAYS 75

CHAPTER ELEVEN 84

Meal Plans and Shopping lists 84

Weekly Meal Plan 84

Grocery Shopping Lists 87

CHAPTER TWELVE 94

Additional Tips for Success 94

Conclusion 97

Introduction

Understanding Stage 4 kidney disease

Chronic Kidney Disease (CKD) affects millions of people worldwide, with varying degrees of severity. It is classified into five stages based on the level of kidney function.

Stage 4 CKD signifies a severe decline in kidney function, with a glomerular filtration rate (GFR) between 15 and 29 milliliters per minute. At this stage, the kidneys are significantly impaired, and patients are often preparing for the possibility of dialysis or a kidney transplant.

The journey through Stage 4 CKD can be challenging, but with the right knowledge and tools, it is possible to manage the condition effectively. One of the most critical aspects of managing Stage 4 CKD is adhering to a kidney-friendly diet.

This cookbook is designed to provide a comprehensive guide to understanding, planning, and preparing meals that support kidney health and enhance your quality of life.

The Importance of Diet in CKD Management

Diet is vital in managing CKD, particularly in its advanced stages. Proper nutrition can help slow the progression of the disease, control symptoms, and improve overall well-being.

For individuals with Stage 4 CKD, dietary choices must be carefully managed to ensure they meet nutritional needs while avoiding substances that can further burden the kidneys.

The primary goals of a Stage 4 kidney diet are to:

1. Limit the intake of certain nutrients such as sodium, potassium, and phosphorus.

2. Control protein consumption to reduce waste buildup in the blood.

3. Maintain adequate calorie intake to prevent malnutrition.

4. Manage fluid intake to avoid fluid overload and swelling.

This cookbook aims to simplify the complexities of a Stage 4 kidney diet, offering practical advice and delicious recipes that align with these nutritional guidelines.

Getting Started with Your Kidney-Friendly Journey

Embarking on a kidney-friendly diet can feel overwhelming, but with the right guidance and resources, it becomes manageable and even enjoyable. This cookbook is structured to provide you with all the information you need to make informed dietary choices.

Here's a glimpse of what you'll find:

Nutritional Guidelines: Clear explanations of the dietary restrictions and recommendations for Stage 4 CKD, including tips for managing protein, sodium, potassium, phosphorus, and fluids.

Meal Planning and Preparation: Practical advice on meal planning, grocery shopping, and cooking techniques to ensure you're well-prepared to follow your kidney-friendly diet.

Delicious Recipes: A wide variety of recipes for breakfast, lunch, dinner, snacks, and desserts that are specifically designed to be kidney-friendly without compromising on taste.

Special Occasions: Ideas for celebrating holidays and special occasions with meals that are both festive and kidney-friendly.

Weekly Meal Plans: Sample meal plans and grocery lists to help you stay organized and maintain a balanced diet.

Your Path to Better Kidney Health

We understand that living with Stage 4 CKD can be daunting, but you are not alone. This cookbook is a resource to empower you with the knowledge and tools needed to manage your condition effectively.

By making thoughtful dietary choices, you can positively impact your health and well-being.

As you explore the recipes and tips within this book, we hope you'll discover that a kidney-friendly diet can be both nutritious and delicious. Remember, every small step you take toward better nutrition is a step toward better kidney health.

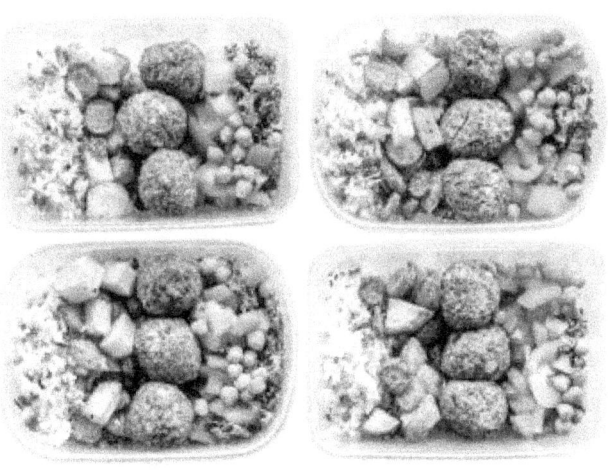

CHAPTER ONE

Overview of Kidney Function

The two bean-shaped organs located on either side of the spine, just below the ribcage are called Kidneys. They perform several vital functions to maintain the body's overall health, including:

Filtration of Blood: The primary function of the kidneys is to filter waste products and excess substances (such as water, electrolytes, and toxins) from the blood to form urine.

Regulation of Fluid and Electrolyte Balance: The kidneys help maintain the right balance of fluids and electrolytes (sodium, potassium, and calcium) in the body.

Acid-Base Balance: They regulate the pH level of the blood by excreting hydrogen ions and reabsorbing bicarbonate from urine.

Blood Pressure Regulation: The kidneys produce an enzyme called renin, which plays a crucial role in regulating blood pressure.

Red Blood Cell Production: They produce erythropoietin, a hormone that stimulates the production of red blood cells in the bone marrow.

Bone Health: The kidneys help activate vitamin D, which is essential for calcium absorption and bone health.

Stages of Chronic Kidney Disease (CKD)

Chronic Kidney Disease (CKD) is a condition in which kidney function gradually declines over time. CKD is divided into five stages based on the glomerular filtration rate (GFR), which measures how well the kidneys filter waste from the blood.

Stage 1 (GFR ≥ 90 mL/min): Kidney damage with normal or increased GFR. There are typically no symptoms, but early signs of kidney damage (such as protein in the urine) may be present.

Stage 2 (GFR 60-89 mL/min): Mild reduction in kidney function. Similar to Stage 1, there are usually no obvious symptoms, but laboratory tests may indicate some kidney damage.

Stage 3 (GFR 30-59 mL/min): Moderate reduction in kidney function. Symptoms such as fatigue, swelling (edema), and changes in urine output may start to appear. This stage is often divided into Stage 3a (GFR 45-59) and Stage 3b (GFR 30-44).

Stage 4 (GFR 15-29 mL/min): Severe reduction in kidney function. Symptoms become more pronounced, and complications such as high blood pressure, anemia, and bone disease may develop. Patients often need to prepare for dialysis or a kidney transplant.

Stage 5 (GFR < 15 mL/min): Kidney failure or end-stage renal disease (ESRD). The kidneys are no longer able to maintain the body's fluid and electrolyte balance, and dialysis or a kidney transplant is required to sustain life.

Specifics of Stage 4 CKD

Stage 4 CKD is characterized by a severe decline in kidney function, with a GFR between 15 and 29 mL/min. At this stage, the kidneys are significantly impaired and unable to adequately filter waste products and excess substances from the blood. Key aspects of Stage 4 CKD include:

Symptoms: Common symptoms include fatigue, swelling (edema) in the hands and feet, shortness of breath, difficulty concentrating, decreased urine output, and changes in urine color.

Complications: Patients may experience complications such as high blood pressure, anemia, bone disease, cardiovascular disease, and electrolyte imbalances (high potassium and phosphorus levels).

Medical Management: Close monitoring and management by a healthcare team are essential. Medications may be prescribed to control blood pressure, manage anemia, and balance electrolytes.

Dietary Restrictions: A carefully managed diet becomes crucial to limit the intake of certain nutrients (such as sodium, potassium, phosphorus, and protein) to reduce the burden on the kidneys.

Preparation for Dialysis or Transplant: Patients often need to begin preparing for the possibility of dialysis or a kidney transplant. This may involve creating a vascular access site for dialysis or undergoing evaluations for transplant eligibility.

Importance of Diet in CKD Management

Diet plays a critical role in managing CKD, especially in its advanced stages. The right dietary choices can help slow the progression of the disease, alleviate symptoms, and prevent complications. Key dietary considerations for CKD management include:

Protein Intake: Controlled protein intake is essential to reduce the buildup of waste products in the blood. High-quality protein sources (such as lean meats, eggs, and dairy) are recommended in limited quantities.

Sodium Restriction: Reducing sodium intake helps manage blood pressure and prevent fluid retention. This involves avoiding processed and salty foods and using herbs and spices for flavoring.

Potassium Management: Maintaining appropriate potassium levels is crucial to prevent hyperkalemia (high potassium levels), which can affect heart function. Foods high in potassium (such as bananas, oranges, and potatoes) should be limited.

Phosphorus Control: Controlling phosphorus intake helps prevent bone disease and cardiovascular complications. Foods high in phosphorus (such as dairy products, nuts, and beans) should be restricted.

Fluid Intake: Monitoring fluid intake is important to prevent fluid overload and swelling. This includes beverages and foods with high water content.

Overall Nutrition: Ensuring adequate calorie intake to maintain a healthy weight and prevent malnutrition is important. Nutrient-dense foods (such as fruits, vegetables, whole grains, and healthy fats) should be included in appropriate portions.

By following these dietary guidelines, individuals with CKD can better manage their condition, improve their quality of life, and reduce the risk of complications.

This cookbook provides practical advice and recipes tailored to meet the unique nutritional needs of those with Stage 4 CKD, helping them navigate their dietary journey with confidence and ease.

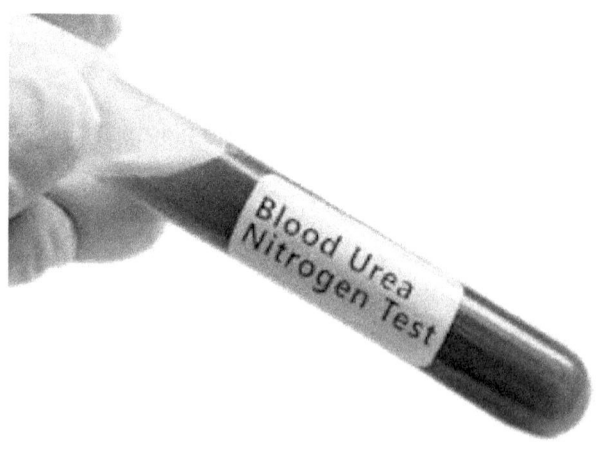

CHAPTER TWO

Nutritional Guidelines for Stage 4 kidney disease

Managing Stage 4 kidney disease requires careful attention to diet to slow the progression of the disease, manage symptoms, and prevent complications. Here are the key nutritional guidelines:

Protein Intake

Why It's Important:

In Stage 4 CKD, the kidneys struggle to filter out waste products from protein metabolism. Controlling protein intake helps reduce this burden.

Guidelines:

Moderate Protein Intake: Aim for about 0.6 to 0.8 grams of protein per kilogram of body weight per day. This helps minimize waste buildup while providing enough protein to maintain muscle mass and overall health.

High-Quality Proteins: Focus on high-quality protein sources that provide essential amino acids, such as lean meats, poultry, fish, eggs, and dairy in controlled amounts.

Plant-Based Proteins: Incorporate plant-based proteins like beans, lentils, and tofu in moderation, as they tend to produce less waste compared to animal proteins.

Sodium Restrictions

Why It's Important:

Excess sodium can lead to high blood pressure and fluid retention, exacerbating kidney disease symptoms and complications.

Guidelines:

Limit Sodium Intake: Aim for less than 2,000 milligrams (mg) of sodium per day.

Avoid Processed Foods: Steer clear of processed and packaged foods, which are often high in sodium. This includes canned soups, frozen dinners, snack foods, and deli meats.

Use Fresh Ingredients: Cook with fresh, whole ingredients and flavor your food with herbs, spices, lemon juice, and vinegar instead of salt.

Read Labels: Pay close attention to food labels and choose low-sodium or no-salt-added versions when available.

Potassium Management

Why It's Important:

High potassium levels (hyperkalemia) can be dangerous and affect heart function. Managing potassium intake is crucial to prevent complications.

Guidelines:

Monitor Potassium Levels: Regularly check your blood potassium levels with your healthcare provider.

Limit High-Potassium Foods: Reduce intake of high-potassium foods such as bananas, oranges, potatoes, tomatoes, spinach, and avocados.

Choose Low-Potassium Alternatives: opt for lower-potassium fruits and vegetables like apples, berries, grapes, cauliflower, and green beans.

Leaching Vegetables: When consuming higher-potassium vegetables, use the leaching method (soaking and boiling) to reduce their potassium content.

Phosphorus Control

Why It's Important:

High phosphorus levels can lead to bone disease and cardiovascular issues. Managing phosphorus intake helps maintain bone health and prevent complications.

Guidelines:

Limit Phosphorus-Rich Foods: Avoid foods high in phosphorus such as dairy products, nuts, seeds, beans, lentils, organ meats, and processed foods with phosphate additives.

Choose Phosphorus Binders: Your healthcare provider may prescribe phosphorus binders to take with meals to help reduce phosphorus absorption.

Read Labels: Be aware of ingredients that contain added phosphates (often listed as "phosphoric acid," "disodium phosphate," etc.) and choose products without these additives.

Fluid Intake Recommendations

Why It's Important:

Proper fluid management helps prevent fluid overload, which can cause swelling, high blood pressure, and difficulty breathing.

Guidelines:

Monitor Fluid Intake: Your healthcare provider will give you a specific fluid allowance based on your individual needs. This includes all liquids (water, coffee, tea, etc.) and foods with high water content (soups, gelatin, ice cream).

Track Fluid Consumption: Keep a daily record of your fluid intake to ensure you stay within your recommended limits.

Control Thirst: Manage thirst with small sips of water, sucking on ice chips, chewing gum, or using hard candy. Avoid salty foods, which can increase thirst.

Weigh Daily: Weigh yourself daily to monitor for sudden increases in weight, which may indicate fluid retention.

By adhering to these nutritional guidelines, individuals with Stage 4 CKD can help manage their condition more effectively and improve their quality of life. This cookbook will provide practical recipes and meal-planning tips to help you follow these dietary recommendations while enjoying delicious and satisfying meals.

CHAPTER THREE

Getting Started

Essential Kitchen Tools

Having the right tools in your kitchen can make preparing kidney-friendly meals easier and more enjoyable. Here are some essentials:

Measuring Cups and Spoons: Precise measurement is crucial for controlling portion sizes and nutrient intake.

Kitchen Scale: Useful for weighing foods to ensure accurate portion control, especially for proteins and high-potassium foods.

Sharp Knives: A good set of knives makes chopping vegetables and other ingredients quicker and safer.

Cutting Boards: Have separate cutting boards for meats and vegetables to avoid cross-contamination.

Non-Stick Cookware: Helps reduce the need for added fats when cooking.

Blender or Food Processor: Great for making smoothies, purees, and soups with controlled **ingredients.**

Steamer Basket: A healthy way to cook vegetables while preserving nutrients.

Slow Cooker or Instant Pot: Convenient for preparing meals in advance and ensuring tender, flavorful dishes.

Storage Containers: For portioning out meals and snacks, making it easier to stick to your dietary plan.

Stocking a Kidney-Friendly Pantry

Keeping your pantry stocked with kidney-friendly foods ensures you always have the ingredients needed for healthy meals. Here are some staples:

Low-Sodium Broths and Soups: For cooking and flavoring dishes without excessive sodium.

Whole Grains: Such as quinoa, barley, and brown rice. These provide fiber and nutrients without high potassium or phosphorus.

Low-Potassium Vegetables: Canned or frozen green beans, carrots, cauliflower, and bell peppers.

Fruits: Fresh or canned in juice, such as apples, berries, and peaches, for snacks and desserts.

High-Quality Protein Sources: Canned tuna or chicken packed in water, dried beans (in moderation), and lentils.

Herbs and Spices: Basil, oregano, garlic powder, onion powder, and other salt-free seasonings.

Healthy Fats: Olive oil, canola oil, and avocado oil for cooking and dressings.

Phosphorus-Free Dairy Alternatives: Almond milk, rice milk, and other plant-based milks without added phosphates.

Meal Planning Tips

Effective meal planning can help you adhere to your dietary restrictions and make healthy eating easier. Here are some tips:

Plan Ahead: Create a weekly meal plan to ensure you have balanced, kidney-friendly meals each day.

Variety: Include a variety of foods to ensure you get a wide range of nutrients and avoid dietary monotony.

Portion Control: Use measuring tools to keep portion sizes in check, especially for high-protein and high-potassium foods.

Prep in Advance: Prepare ingredients or meals ahead of time to save time during busy days and reduce the temptation to eat unhealthy foods.

Incorporate Leftovers: Plan meals that can use leftovers creatively to minimize waste and effort.

Stay Flexible: Allow for some flexibility in your meal plan to accommodate changes in appetite or availability of ingredients.

Reading Food Labels

Reading food labels is essential for managing sodium, potassium, and phosphorus intake. Here's how to do it effectively:

Check Serving Sizes: Ensure the serving size on the label matches the amount you plan to eat.

Sodium Content: Look for foods with less than 140 mg of sodium per serving to help stay within your daily limit.

Potassium and Phosphorus: Not all labels list these nutrients, but check for foods specifically marked as low in potassium or phosphorus.

Ingredient List: Avoid products with added phosphates (often listed as "phosphoric acid," "disodium phosphate," etc.). Look for hidden sources of sodium like sodium nitrate, sodium benzoate, and monosodium glutamate (MSG).

Health Claims: Be cautious of claims like "low-sodium" or "reduced sodium," and always check the actual numbers on the nutrition label.

Added Sugars: Check for added sugars and opt for products with minimal or no added sugars to maintain overall health.

By equipping your kitchen with the right tools, stocking it with kidney-friendly staples, planning meals thoughtfully, and reading food labels carefully, you'll be well-prepared to follow a diet that supports your kidney health. This cookbook will provide you with delicious recipes and practical advice to make these guidelines easy to follow and enjoyable

CHAPTER FOUR

Breakfast Recipes

Nutritious Breakfast Options

Starting your day with a nutritious and kidney-friendly breakfast sets the tone for making healthy choices throughout the day. Here are some delicious and easy-to-prepare breakfast recipes that align with the dietary restrictions of Stage 4 CKD.

1. Low-Sodium Oatmeal with Fresh Berries

Ingredients:

1 cup water or low-sodium almond milk

1/2 cup old-fashioned rolled oats

1/4 cup fresh berries (blueberries, strawberries, raspberries)

1/2 teaspoon cinnamon

1 tablespoon honey or maple syrup (optional)

A pinch of salt (optional and minimal)

Preparation

Boil Liquid: In a small saucepan, bring the water or low-sodium almond milk to a boil.

Cook Oats: Add the oats, reduce heat to medium, and cook for about 5-7 minutes, stirring occasionally until the oats are soft and the liquid is absorbed.

Add Flavor: Stir in the cinnamon and honey or maple syrup if using.

Top with Berries: Transfer the oatmeal to a bowl and top with fresh berries.

Serve: Enjoy your low-sodium oatmeal warm.

Nutritional Benefits:

Oats: High in fiber and helps maintain stable blood sugar levels.

Berries: Packed with antioxidants and vitamins while being low in potassium.

2. Veggie Omelet with Bell Peppers and Spinach

Ingredients:

Two large eggs or Half a cup of egg substitute

1/4 cup chopped bell peppers (red, green, or yellow)

1/4 cup fresh spinach, chopped

1/4 cup diced onions (optional)

1 tablespoon olive oil or cooking spray

Salt and pepper to taste (minimal salt)

Fresh herbs (parsley, chives) for garnish

Preparation

Prep Vegetables: Chop the bell peppers, spinach, and onions if using.

Heat Pan: Heat the olive oil in a non-stick skillet over medium heat.

Cook Veggies: Add the bell peppers and onions to the skillet and cook for 3-4 minutes until they begin to soften. Add the spinach and cook for another 1-2 minutes until wilted.

Beat Eggs: In a small bowl, beat the eggs and season with minimal salt and pepper.

Cook Eggs: Pour the eggs into the skillet with the vegetables. Cook until the eggs begin to set, then gently lift the edges to let uncooked eggs flow underneath.

Fold Omelet: Once the omelet is fully set, fold it in half and cook for an additional minute.

Garnish and Serve: Garnish with fresh herbs and serve warm.

Nutritional Benefits:

Eggs: Provide high-quality protein without overburdening the kidneys.

Vegetables: Low in potassium and add vitamins and minerals.

3. Smoothies with Kidney-Friendly Ingredients

Ingredients:

1/2 cup fresh or frozen berries (blueberries, strawberries, raspberries)

1/2 cup almond milk or coconut milk (low in potassium and phosphorus)

1/2 cup Greek yogurt (low in phosphorus and potassium)

1 tablespoon chia seeds (optional)

1 tablespoon honey or maple syrup (optional)

A handful of fresh spinach (optional)

Preparation

Combine Ingredients: Add all the ingredients to a blender.

Blend: Blend on high until smooth and creamy. If the smoothie is too thick, then add extra almond milk.

Serve: Immediately pour into a glass and enjoy.

Nutritional Benefits:

Berries and **Spinach:** Provide antioxidants and essential vitamins with minimal potassium.

Greek Yogurt: Offers a good source of protein and probiotics without high phosphorus levels.

Chia Seeds: Add fiber and omega-3 fatty acids, beneficial for heart health.

4. Whole Grain Toast with Avocado Spread

Ingredients:

1 slice whole grain bread (low-sodium)

1/2 ripe avocado

1 teaspoon lemon juice

Salt and pepper to taste (minimal salt)

Optional toppings: cherry tomatoes, radishes, fresh herbs

Preparation.

Toast Bread: Toast the whole grain bread to your

desired level of crispiness.

Prepare Avocado Spread: In a small bowl, mash the avocado with a fork. Mix in the lemon juice and season with minimal salt and pepper.

Spread Avocado: Spread the avocado mixture evenly over the toast.

Add Toppings: Add optional toppings like sliced cherry tomatoes, radishes, or fresh herbs for extra flavor and nutrition.

Serve: Enjoy immediately.

Nutritional Benefits:

Whole Grain Bread: Provides fiber and nutrients without high sodium.

Avocado: Offers healthy fats and vitamins wIth controlled potassium.

These breakfast options are tailored to provide balanced nutrition while adhering to the dietary restrictions of Stage 4 CKD. They are easy to prepare, delicious, and packed with essential nutrients to help you start your day right.

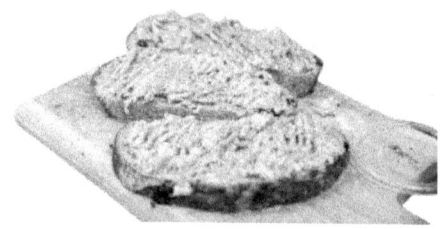

Whole Grain Toast with Avocado Spread

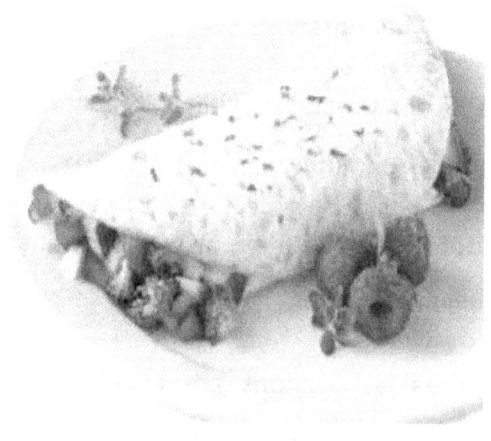

. Veggie Omelet with Bell Peppers and Spinach

CHAPTER FIVE

Lunch Recipes

Healthy Lunch Ideas

A nutritious and balanced lunch can provide sustained energy and keep you feeling satisfied throughout the afternoon. Here are some kidney-friendly lunch recipes that are both delicious and easy to prepare.

1. Quinoa Salad with Cucumber and Mint

Ingredients:

- 1 cup quinoa, rinsed

- 2 cups water

- 1 cup cucumber, diced

- 1/4 cup fresh mint leaves, chopped

- 1/4 cup red bell pepper, diced

- 1/4 cup red onion, finely chopped

- 2 tablespoons olive oil

- 2 tablespoons lemon juice

- Salt and pepper to taste (minimal salt)

Preparation.

Cook Quinoa: Bring the water to a boil In a medium saucepan. Add the quinoa, reduce the heat to low, cover, and simmer for about 15 minutes or until the quinoa is tender and the water is absorbed. Remove from heat and let cool.

Prepare Vegetables: While the quinoa is cooling, dice the cucumber, bell pepper, and red onion. Chop the mint leaves.

Mix Salad: In a large bowl, combine the cooled quinoa, cucumber, mint, bell pepper, and red onion.

Dress Salad: In a small bowl, whisk together the olive oil, lemon juice, and a pinch of salt and pepper. After adding the dressing to the salad, toss to mix.

Serve: Serve either room temperature or cold.

Nutritional Benefits:

Quinoa: A good source of plant-based protein and fiber.

Vegetables: Provide vitamins, minerals, and antioxidants with minimal potassium.

2. Grilled Chicken Wrap with Low-Sodium Hummus

Ingredients:

- 1 whole wheat tortilla

- 1 small chicken breast, grilled and sliced

- 2 tablespoons low-sodium hummus

- 1/4 cup shredded lettuce

- 1/4 cup sliced cucumber

- 1/4 cup shredded carrots

- 1 tablespoon olive oil

- Salt and pepper to taste (minimal salt)

Preparation.

Grill Chicken: Season the chicken breast with a minimal amount of salt and pepper. Grill over medium heat for about 6-7 minutes per side or until fully cooked. Let cool and slice thinly.

Prepare Wrap: Spread the low-sodium hummus evenly over the whole wheat tortilla.

Add Ingredients: Layer the grilled chicken slices, shredded lettuce, sliced cucumber, and shredded carrots on top of the hummus.

Roll and Serve Roll up the tortilla tightly and cut in half. Serve immediately.

Nutritional Benefits:

Chicken: Provides high-quality protein with low sodium.

Vegetables: Add crunch and nutrients without high potassium.

3. Kidney-Friendly Vegetable Soup

Ingredients:

- 1 tablespoon olive oil

- 1 small onion, chopped

- 2 cloves garlic, minced

- 2 carrots, diced

- 2 celery stalks, diced

- 1 zucchini, diced

-A cup green beans, trimmed and cut into 1-inch pieces

- 4 cups low-sodium vegetable broth

- one can (14.5 ounces) no-salt-added diced tomatoes

- 1 teaspoon dried thyme

- 1 teaspoon dried basil

- Salt and pepper to taste (minimal salt)

Preparation:

Sauté Vegetables: Heat the olive oil In a large saucepan over medium heat. Add the onion and garlic, and sauté until softened, about 5 minutes.

Add Broth and Vegetables: Add the carrots, celery, zucchini, green beans, and low-sodium vegetable broth. After bringing to a boil, lower heat, and simmer for roughly 20 minutes.

Add Tomatoes and Seasonings: Stir in the diced tomatoes, thyme, and basil. Season with a small amount of salt and pepper. Simmer for another ten to fifteen minutes, or until the vegetables are soft.

Serve: Ladle the soup into bowls and serve warm.

Nutritional Benefits:

Vegetables Provide fiber, vitamins, and minerals with low potassium and sodium.

Low-Sodium Broth: Reduces overall sodium intake while adding flavor.

4. Tuna Salad with Greek Yogurt Dressing

Ingredients

1 can (5 ounces) tuna packed in water, drained

1/4 cup plain Greek yogurt

1 tablespoon lemon juice

1 tablespoon Dijon mustard

1 celery stalk, diced

1/4 cup red bell pepper, diced

2 tablespoons red onion, finely chopped

1 tablespoon fresh parsley, chopped

Salt and pepper to taste (minimal salt)

Lettuce leaves or whole grain crackers for serving

Preparation.

Mix Dressing: In a medium bowl, combine the Greek yogurt, lemon juice, and Dijon mustard.

Prepare Tuna Salad: Add the drained tuna, diced celery, red bell pepper, red onion, and parsley to the bowl. Mix until well combined.

Season: Season with a minimal amount of salt and pepper to taste.

Serve: Serve the tuna salad on whole grain crackers or in lettuce leaves.

Nutritional Benefits:

Tuna: A good source of lean protein and omega-3 fatty acids.

Greek Yogurt: Adds creaminess with less phosphorus and potassium compared to mayonnaise.

These lunch recipes provide balanced nutrition while adhering to the dietary restrictions necessary for Stage 4 CKD. They are easy to prepare and offer a variety of flavors and textures to keep your meals interesting and satisfying.

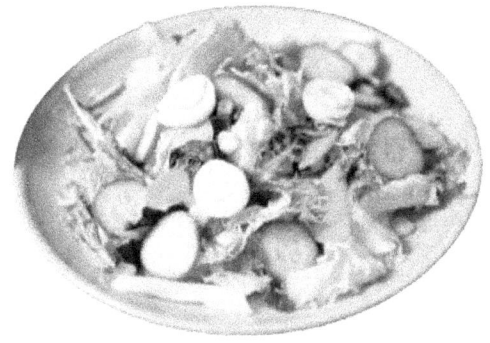

Quinoa Salad with Cucumber and Mint

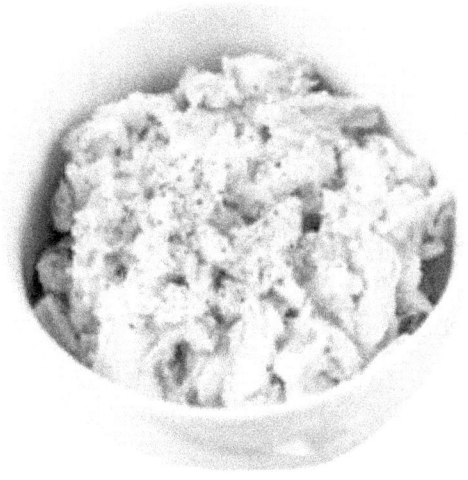

Tuna Salad with Greek Yogurt Dressing

CHAPTER SIX

Dinner Recipes

Satisfying Dinner Choices

A satisfying and well-balanced dinner is crucial for maintaining energy levels and ensuring a restful night's sleep. Here are some kidney-friendly dinner recipes that are both nutritious and delicious.

1. Baked Salmon with Lemon and Dill

Ingredients:

4 salmon fillets (4-6 ounces each)

2 tablespoons olive oil

2 lemons, thinly sliced

2 tablespoons fresh dill, chopped

Salt and pepper to taste (minimal salt)

1 teaspoon garlic powder

Preparation.

Preheat Oven: Preheat the oven to 190°C

Prepare Baking Sheet: Place baking sheet with parchment paper or aluminum foil.

Season Salmon: Place the salmon fillets on the prepared baking sheet. Drizzle with olive oil and season with garlic powder, a minimal amount of salt, and pepper. Top each fillet with lemon slices and drizzle with fresh dill.

Bake Salmon: Bake for 15-20 minutes, or until the salmon is cooked through and flakes easily with a fork.

Serve: Serve the baked salmon with a side of steamed vegetables or a fresh salad.

Nutritional Benefits:

Salmon: Provides high-quality protein and omega-3 fatty acids beneficial for heart health.

Lemon and Dill: Add flavor without adding sodium.

2. Herb-Roasted Chicken with Steamed Vegetables

Ingredients:

4 chicken breasts, bone-in and skin-on

2 tablespoons olive oil

2 teaspoons dried thyme

2 teaspoons dried rosemary

2 teaspoons dried oregano

Salt and pepper to taste (minimal salt)

2 cups mixed vegetables (e.g., broccoli, carrots, cauliflower), steamed

Preparation.

Preheat Oven: Preheat the oven to 200°C.

Prepare Chicken: In a small bowl, mix the olive oil, thyme, rosemary, oregano, and a minimal amount of salt and pepper. Over the chicken breasts, evenly rub the mixture in.

Roast Chicken: Place the chicken breasts on a baking sheet and roast in the oven for 35-40 minutes, or until the chicken is fully cooked and the skin is golden brown.

Steam Vegetables: While the chicken is roasting, steam the mixed vegetables until tender.

Serve: Serve the herb-roasted chicken with a side of steamed vegetables.

Nutritional Benefits:

Chicken: A lean protein source.

Herbs: Enhance flavor without adding sodium.

Steamed Vegetables: Provide essential vitamins and minerals with minimal potassium.

3. Beef Stir-Fry with Bell Peppers and Broccoli

Ingredients:

1-pound lean beef strips

1 tablespoon olive oil

1 red bell pepper, sliced

1 green bell pepper, sliced

1 cup broccoli florets

2 cloves garlic, minced

1 tablespoon low-sodium soy sauce

1 tablespoon fresh ginger, grated

1 tablespoon cornstarch

1/4 cup water

Cooked brown rice for serving

Preparation.

Prepare Beef: In a bowl, toss the beef strips with cornstarch until evenly coated.

Heat Oil: In a large skillet or wok, heat the olive oil over medium-high heat.

Cook Beef: Add the beef strips and cook for 4-5 minutes, or until browned. Remove from the skillet then set aside.

Stir-Fry Vegetables: In the same skillet, add the garlic, ginger, bell peppers, and broccoli. Stir-fry for five to seven minutes, or until the vegetables are tender-crisp.

Combine Ingredients: Return the beef to the skillet. Add the low-sodium soy sauce and water, and stir to combine. Cook for an additional 2-3 minutes.

Serve: Serve the beef stir-fry over cooked brown rice.

Nutritional Benefits:

Beef: Provides high-quality protein and iron.

Bell Peppers and Broccoli: Add vitamins, fiber, and antioxidants with controlled potassium levels.

Low-Sodium Soy Sauce: Reduces sodium intake.

4. Lentil and Vegetable Stew

Ingredients:

1 cup dried lentils, rinsed

1 tablespoon olive oil

1 large onion, chopped

2 carrots, diced

2 celery stalks, diced

2 cloves garlic, minced

1 can (14.5 ounces) no-salt-added diced tomatoes

4 cups low-sodium vegetable broth

1 teaspoon dried thyme

1 teaspoon dried basil

1 bay leaf

Salt and pepper to taste (minimal salt)

Preparation

Sauté Vegetables: Heat the olive oil In a large pot over medium heat. Add the onion, carrots, celery, and garlic, and sauté until the vegetables are softened, about 5 minutes.

Add Ingredients: Stir in the lentils, diced tomatoes, vegetable broth, thyme, basil, and bay leaf. add a small amount of salt and pepper.

Simmer Stew: Bring the mixture to a boil, then reduce heat and simmer for 30-35 minutes, or until the lentils are tender.

Serve: Remove the bay leaf and serve the stew warm.

Nutritional Benefits:

Lentils: Provide plant-based protein and fiber.

Vegetables: Add essential vitamins and minerals without high potassium.

Low-Sodium Broth: Keeps sodium levels in check while adding flavor.

These dinner recipes are designed to be nutritious, satisfying, and suitable for those managing Stage 4 CKD. They offer a variety of flavors and textures to keep meals enjoyable and health-focused.

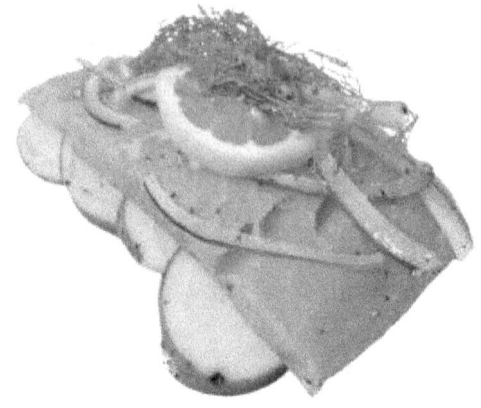

Baked Salmon with Lemon and Dill

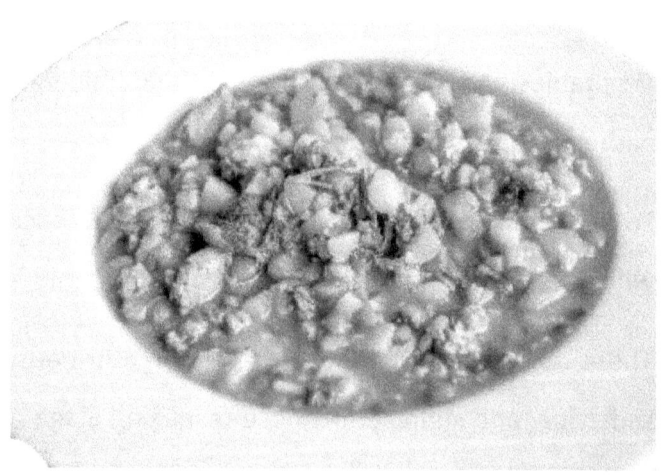

. Lentil and Vegetable Stew

CHAPTER SEVEN

Snack and Side Dish Recipes

Tasty Snacks and Sides

Including healthy snacks and side dishes in your meal plan can help manage hunger between meals and ensure a balanced intake of nutrients. Here are some kidney-friendly options that are easy to prepare and enjoy.

1. Low-Sodium Crackers with Cottage Cheese

Ingredients:

1 cup low-sodium crackers

1/2 cup low-fat cottage cheese

Fresh herbs such as chives or parsley (for garnish)

A pinch of black pepper

Preparation.

Prepare Crackers: Arrange the low-sodium crackers on a serving plate.

Top with Cottage Cheese: Spoon a small amount of low-fat cottage cheese onto each cracker.

Garnish: Sprinkle with fresh herbs and a pinch of black pepper.

Serve: Enjoy immediately as a quick and protein-rich snack.

Nutritional Benefits:

Cottage Cheese: Provides protein with controlled phosphorus levels.

Low-Sodium Crackers: Offers a crunchy texture without adding excessive sodium.

2. Carrot and Cucumber Sticks with Yogurt Dip

Ingredients:

2 large carrots, peeled and cut into sticks

1 large cucumber, cut into sticks

1 cup plain Greek yogurt

1 tablespoon lemon juice

1 teaspoon garlic powder

1 teaspoon dried dill

Salt and pepper to taste (minimal salt)

Preparation.

Prepare Vegetables: Cut the carrots and cucumber into sticks and arrange them on a serving platter.

Make Yogurt Dip: In a small bowl, mix the Greek yogurt, lemon juice, garlic powder, dried dill, and a minimal amount of salt and pepper.

Serve: Serve the vegetable sticks with the yogurt dip.

Nutritional Benefits:

Vegetables: Low in potassium and calories, high in vitamins and fiber.

Greek Yogurt: Adds protein and a creamy texture without excessive sodium.

3. Roasted Cauliflower with Garlic

Ingredients:

1 head of cauliflower, cut into florets

2 tablespoons olive oil

3 cloves garlic, minced

1 teaspoon dried thyme

Salt and pepper to taste (minimal salt)

Fresh parsley for garnish (optional)

Preparation.

Preheat Oven: Preheat the oven to 200°C (400°F).

Prepare Cauliflower: In a large bowl, toss the cauliflower florets with olive oil, minced garlic, dried thyme, and a minimal amount of salt and pepper.

Roast: Spread the cauliflower on a baking sheet in a single layer. Roast for twenty to twenty-five minutes, or until the cauliflower is soft and golden brown, stirring halfway through.

Garnish and Serve: Garnish with fresh parsley if desired and serve warm.

Nutritional Benefits:

Cauliflower: A low-potassium vegetable that adds fiber and vitamins.

Olive Oil: Provides healthy fats for heart health.

4. Apple Slices with Almond Butter

Ingredients:

2 medium apples, cored and sliced

1/4 cup almond butter (unsweetened and unsalted)

A sprinkle of cinnamon (optional)

Preparation

Prepare Apples: Core and slice the apples into thin wedges.

Serve with Almond Butter: Arrange the apple slices on a plate and serve with a small dish of almond butter for dipping.

Optional: Sprinkle a bit of cinnamon over the apple slices for added flavor.

Nutritional Benefits:

Apples: Low in potassium and provide fiber and vitamins.

Almond Butter: Offers healthy fats and protein, with controlled sodium and phosphorus.

These snacks and sides are designed to be nutritious, easy to prepare, and suitable for those managing Stage 4 CKD. They offer a variety of flavors and textures to keep your diet enjoyable and health-focused.

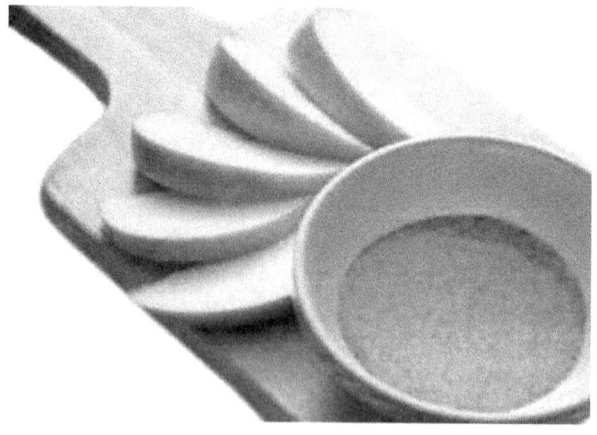

CHAPTER EIGHT

Dessert Recipes

Kidney-Friendly Desserts

Enjoying a delicious dessert while managing Stage 4 CKD is possible with the right ingredients and recipes. Here are some kidney-friendly desserts that are both satisfying and nutritious.

1. Berry Parfait with Greek Yogurt

Ingredients:

1 cup plain Greek yogurt (low-fat)

1/2 cup fresh berries (blueberries, strawberries, raspberries)

1 tablespoon honey or maple syrup (optional)

1/4 cup granola (low-sodium)

Fresh mint leaves for garnish (optional)

Preparation

Layer Ingredients: In a glass or bowl, layer half of the Greek yogurt, followed by half of the berries, a drizzle of honey or maple syrup (if using), and a sprinkle of granola.

Repeat Layers: Repeat the layers with the remaining yogurt, berries, and granola.

Garnish: Top with fresh mint leaves if desired.

Serve: Serve immediately or chill for a more refreshing dessert.

Nutritional Benefits:

Greek Yogurt: Provides protein and probiotics with controlled phosphorus.

Berries: Low in potassium and high in antioxidants.

Granola: Adds a crunchy texture and fiber.

2. Cinnamon-Spiced Apples

Ingredients:

Two medium apples, peeled, cored, and sliced

1 tablespoon lemon juice

1 teaspoon ground cinnamon

1 tablespoon honey or maple syrup

1 tablespoon water

Preparation:

Prepare Apples: Peel, core, then slice the apples.

Cook Apples: In a medium saucepan, combine the apple slices, lemon juice, cinnamon, honey or maple syrup, and water. Cook over medium heat, stirring occasionally, until the apples are tender and slightly caramelized, about 10-15 minutes.

Serve: Serve warm as a comforting dessert.

Nutritional Benefits:

Apples: Low in potassium and provide fiber and

vitamins.

Cinnamon: Adds flavor without adding sodium or sugar.

3. Rice Pudding with Vanilla

Ingredients:

1/2 cup white rice

2 cups water

2 cups low-fat milk or almond milk

1/4 cup sugar

1 teaspoon vanilla extract

A pinch of ground nutmeg (optional)

Fresh berries for garnish (optional)

Preparation:

Cook Rice: In a medium saucepan, bring the water to a boil. Add the rice, reduce heat to low, cover, and simmer until the rice is tender and water is absorbed, about 15-20 minutes.

Add sugar and milk: Whisk in the milk and sugar. Cook over medium heat, stirring frequently, until the mixture thickens and becomes creamy, about 20-25 minutes.

Add Flavoring: Remove from heat and stir in the vanilla extract and nutmeg if using.

Serve: Serve warm or chilled, garnished with fresh berries if desired.

Nutritional Benefits:

Rice: Provides a low-potassium, low-phosphorus carbohydrate source.

Milk: Adds creaminess and calcium with controlled potassium and phosphorus.

4. Lemon Sorbet

Ingredients:

A cup water

A cup sugar

A cup of fresh lemon juice (about 4-6 lemons)

1 tablespoon lemon zest

Preparation:

Make Simple Syrup: In a small saucepan, combine the water and sugar. Over medium heat, bring to a boil and continue to stir until the sugar is dissolved. Remove from heat and let cool.

Combine Ingredients: In a mixing bowl, combine the cooled simple syrup, lemon juice, and lemon zest.

Freeze Mixture: Pour the mixture into an ice cream maker and freeze according to the manufacturer's instructions. Alternatively, pour into a shallow dish and freeze, stirring every 30 minutes until it reaches a sorbet-like consistency.

Serve: Serve the lemon sorbet in small bowls or cups.

Nutritional Benefits:

Lemon: Low in potassium and adds a refreshing

flavor.

Simple Syrup: Provides sweetness without adding excessive calories.

These kidney-friendly desserts are designed to be both delicious and suitable for those managing Stage 4 CKD. They offer a variety of flavors and textures to satisfy your sweet tooth while keeping your diet health-focused.

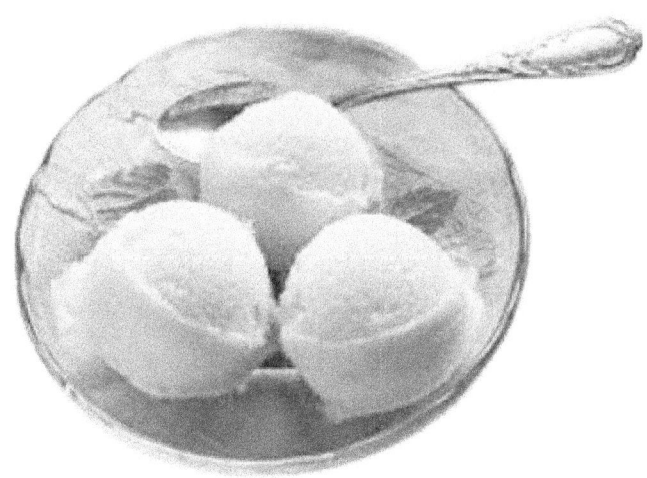

Lemon sorbet

CHAPTER NINE

Beverages

Safe and Refreshing Drinks

Staying hydrated is essential for everyone, including those managing Stage 4 CKD. Choosing the right beverages can help you enjoy refreshing drinks while adhering to your dietary restrictions. Here are some kidney-friendly beverage options.

1. Herbal Teas

Ingredients:

1 teaspoon dried herbs (e.g., chamomile, peppermint, hibiscus)

1 cup boiling water

Lemon slices or a drizzle of honey (optional)

Preparation:

Brew Tea: Place the dried herbs in a tea infuser or

or directly into a cup. Pour boiling water over the herbs and let it soak for five to ten minutes.

Strain and Servet: If not using an infuser, strain the tea to remove the herbs. Add a lemon slice or a drizzle of honey if desired.

Serve: Enjoy warm or over ice for a refreshing iced tea.

Nutritional Benefits:

Herbal Teas: Naturally caffeine-free and low in potassium and phosphorus.

Lemon and Honey: Add flavor without excessive calories or sodium.

2. Infused Water Recipes

Ingredients:

1 liter water

Combinations of fresh fruits, vegetables, and herbs (e.g., cucumber and mint, lemon and lime, strawberry and basil)

Preparation:

Prepare Ingredients: Wash and slice the fruits and vegetables. Tear the herbs slightly to release their flavors.

Combine and Chill: In a large pitcher, combine the water and the chosen ingredients. Let it sit in the refrigerator for at least 120 minutes to allow the flavors to infuse.

Serve: Serve chilled, with or without the added ingredients.

Nutritional Benefits:

Infused Water: Enhances hydration with natural flavors without adding calories, potassium, or sodium.

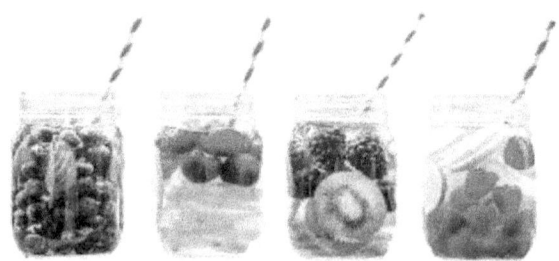

3. Smoothies with Controlled Potassium Levels

Ingredients:

Half a cup of frozen berries (strawberries, blueberries, or raspberries)

1/2 cup unsweetened almond milk or low-fat milk

1/4 cup plain Greek yogurt

1 tablespoon flaxseed or chia seeds

1 teaspoon honey or maple syrup (optional)

Preparation:

Blend Ingredients: Combine all ingredients in a blender and blend until smooth.

Adjust Consistency: If the smoothie is too thick, add a little more almond milk or water until the desired consistency is reached.

Serve: Pour into a glass and serve immediately.

Nutritional Benefits:

Berries: Low in potassium and high in antioxidants.

Greek Yogurt: Adds protein with controlled phosphorus levels.

Almond Milk: Low in potassium and phosphorus compared to cow's milk.

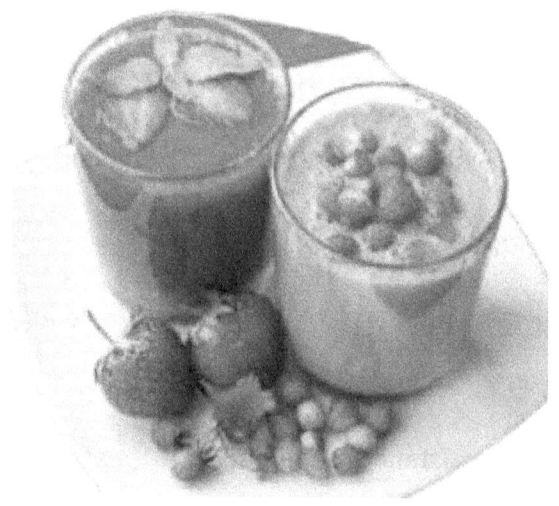

4. Low-Sodium Broths

Ingredients:

4 cups low-sodium vegetable, chicken, or beef broth

Fresh herbs (such as parsley, thyme, or rosemary) for added flavor

Preparation:

Heat Broth: In a medium saucepan, heat the low-sodium broth over medium heat until hot.

Add Herbs: Add fresh herbs to the broth for additional flavor.

Serve: Serve warm in a cup or bowl.

Nutritional Benefits:

Low-Sodium Broth: Provides hydration and electrolytes with minimal sodium.

Herbs: Enhance flavor without adding sodium.

These beverages offer a variety of refreshing and nutritious options for those managing Stage 4 CKD.

They are designed to keep you hydrated and satisfied while adhering to dietary restrictions

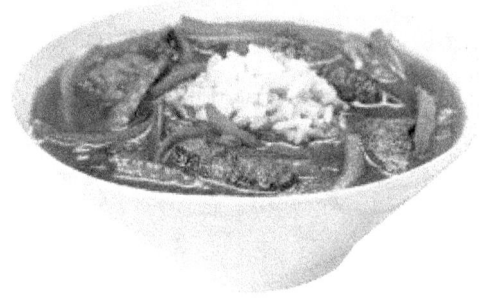

Low sodium Beef Broth

CHAPTER TEN

SPECIAL OCCASIONS AND HOLIDAYS

Festive and Special Occasion Meals

Celebrating special occasions and holidays with loved ones can be enjoyable and healthy, even while managing Stage 4 CKD. Here are some kidney-friendly recipes for festive meals, birthday treats, and picnic or barbecue gatherings.

1. Kidney-Friendly Holiday Feast

Main Course: Herb-Crusted Turkey Breast

Ingredients:

1 turkey breast (about 3-4 pounds)

2 tablespoons olive oil

1 tablespoon dried rosemary

1 tablespoon dried thyme

1 tablespoon dried sage

3 cloves garlic, minced

Salt and pepper to taste (minimal salt)

Preparation

Preheat Oven: Preheat the oven to 175°C (350°F)

Prepare Turkey: In a small bowl, mix the olive oil, rosemary, thyme, sage, minced garlic, and a minimal amount of salt and pepper. evenly apply the mixture all over the turkey breast.

Roast Turkey: Place the turkey breast on a roasting pan and roast in the oven for 1.5 to 2 hours, or until the internal temperature reaches 165°F (75°C). Before slicing., Let it sit for ten minutes

Serve: Serve with kidney-friendly side dishes like steamed green beans or roasted carrots.

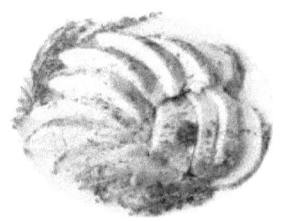

2. Side Dish: Mashed Cauliflower

Ingredients:

1 head cauliflower, cut into florets

1/4 cup low-fat milk or unsweetened almond milk

2 tablespoons olive oil

2 cloves garlic, minced

Salt and pepper to taste (minimal salt)

Preparation:

Steam Cauliflower: Steam the cauliflower florets until tender, about 10-15 minutes.

Blend: In a food processor or blender, combine the steamed cauliflower, milk, olive oil, minced garlic, and a minimal amount of salt and pepper. Blend until smooth and creamy.

Serve: Serve warm as a healthy alternative to mashed potatoes.

3. Birthday Treats

Dessert: Strawberry Shortcake

Ingredients:

1 cup all-purpose flour

1/4 cup sugar

1 teaspoon baking powder

1/4 teaspoon salt

1/4 cup cold unsalted butter, cubed

1/4 cup low-fat milk

1 teaspoon vanilla extract

1 cup fresh strawberries, sliced

1 cup plain Greek yogurt (for topping)

1 tablespoon honey (optional)

Preparation

Preheat Oven: Preheat the oven to 200°C (400°F).

Prepare Shortcake Dough: In a mixing bowl, combine the flour, sugar, baking powder, and salt. Add the chilled butter and stir until the mixture resembles coarse crumbs. Whisk in the milk and vanilla extract until just combined.

Bake: Drop spoonful of the dough onto a baking sheet and bake for 12-15 minutes or until golden brown. Let cool.

Assemble Shortcake: Slice the shortcakes in half. Top the bottom half with sliced strawberries and a dollop of Greek yogurt sweetened with honey (if using). Place the second half on top and serve.

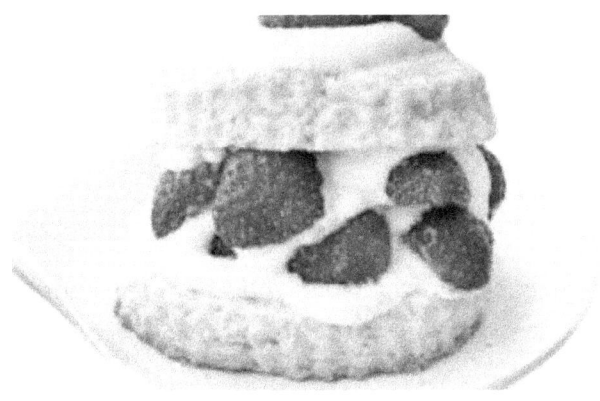

4. Picnic and Barbecue Ideas

Main Dish: Grilled Chicken Skewers

Ingredients:

1 pound chicken breast, cut into cubes

2 tablespoons olive oil

1 teaspoon dried oregano

1 teaspoon dried basil

1 teaspoon garlic powder

1 red bell pepper, cut into chunks

1 green bell pepper, cut into chunks

1 red onion, cut into chunks

Salt and pepper to taste (minimal salt)

Preparation:

Prepare Marinade: In a bowl, mix the olive oil, oregano, basil, garlic powder, and a minimal amount of salt and pepper. Add the chicken cubes then marinate for at least thirty minutes.

Assemble Skewers: Thread the chicken cubes, bell peppers, and red onion onto skewers.

Grill: Preheat the grill to medium-high heat. Grill the skewers for ten to twelve minutes, turning occasionally, till the chicken is cooked through.

Serve: Serve with a side of mixed greens or a kidney-friendly pasta salad.

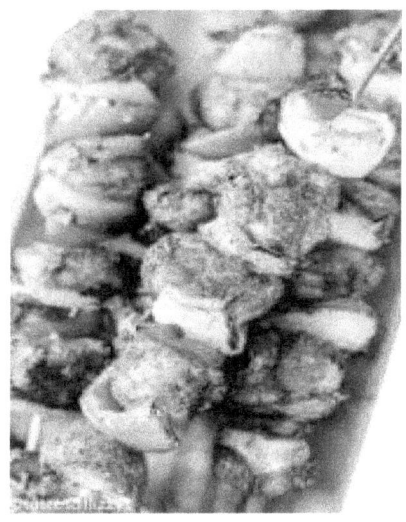

5. Side Dish: Quinoa Salad

Ingredients:

1 cup quinoa, rinsed

2 cups water

1 cup cherry tomatoes, halved

1 cucumber, diced

1/4 cup fresh parsley, chopped

2 tablespoons olive oil

1 tablespoon lemon juice

Salt and pepper to taste (minimal salt)

Preparation:

Cook Quinoa: In a saucepan, bring the water to a boil. Add the quinoa, reduce heat to low, cover, and simmer for 15 minutes, or until the water is absorbed. Let cool.

Prepare Salad: In a large bowl, combine the cooked quinoa, cherry tomatoes, cucumber, and parsley.

Make Dressing: In a small bowl, whisk together the olive oil, lemon juice, and a minimal amount of salt and pepper. Pour over the salad then toss to mix

Serve: Serve chilled or at room temperature.

These recipes are designed to help you celebrate special occasions and holidays with delicious, kidney-friendly meals that everyone can enjoy. Whether it's a holiday feast, a birthday treats, or a picnic gathering, these options ensure you can participate in the festivities while managing Stage 4 CKD.

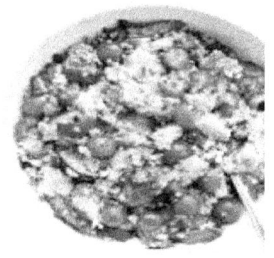

CHAPTER ELEVEN

Meal Plans and Shopping lists

Weekly Meal Plan

Day 1

Breakfast: Greek yogurt with honey and mixed berries

Lunch: Grilled chicken salad with avocado and balsamic vinaigrette dressing

Dinner: Baked salmon with quinoa and steamed broccoli

Snack: Apple slices with almond butter

Day 2

Breakfast: Oatmeal with bananas and chia seeds

Lunch: On whole grain bread, a turkey and cheese sandwich are served with a side salad.

Dinner: marinara sauced spaghetti served with garlic bread on the side

Snack: Carrot sticks with hummus

Day 3

Breakfast: Spinach, banana, and protein powder smoothie

Lunch: Quinoa salad with cucumber, feta, and chickpeas

Dinner: Chicken stir-fry with bell peppers and brown rice

Snack: Mixed nuts

Day 4

Breakfast: Scrambled eggs with spinach and tomatoes

Lunch: Lentil soup and whole grain bread

Dinner: Beef tacos with lettuce, cheese, and salsa

Snack: Greek yogurt with granola

Day 5

Breakfast: Poached eggs, avocado, and whole grain bread

Lunch: Caesar salad with grilled shrimp

Dinner: Baked chicken thighs with roasted sweet potatoes and green beans

Snack: Cottage cheese with pineapple

Day 6

Breakfast: Pancakes with fresh berries and maple syrup

Lunch: Veggie wrap with hummus, cucumber, and bell peppers

Dinner: Grilled steak mashed potatoes and asparagus

Snack: Fruit smoothie

Day 7

Breakfast: Bagel with cream cheese and smoked salmon

Lunch: Chicken Caesar wrap

Dinner: Vegetable lasagna

Snack: Dark chocolate and almonds

Grocery Shopping Lists

Day 1

Greek yogurt

Honey

Mixed berries

Chicken breast

Avocado

Mixed greens

Balsamic vinaigrette

Salmon fillets

Quinoa

Broccoli

Apples

Almond butter

Day 2

Oatmeal

Bananas

Chia seeds

Turkey slices

Cheese

Whole grain bread

Salad greens

Spaghetti

Marinara sauce

Garlic bread

Carrots

Hummus

Day 3

Spinach

Bananas

Protein powder

Quinoa

Chickpeas

Cucumber

Feta cheese

Chicken breast

Bell peppers

Brown rice

Mixed nuts

Day 4

Eggs

Spinach

Tomatoes

Lentils

Whole grain bread

Ground beef

Taco shells

Lettuce

Cheese

Salsa

Greek yogurt

Granola

Day 5

Whole grain bread

Avocado

Eggs

Romaine lettuce

Shrimp

Chicken thighs

Sweet potatoes

Green beans

Cottage cheese

Pineapple

Day 6

Pancake mix

Fresh berries

Maple syrup

Whole grain wrap

Hummus

Cucumber

Bell peppers

Steak

Potatoes

Asparagus

Frozen fruit (for smoothies)

Day 7

Bagels

Cream cheese

Smoked salmon

Chicken breast

Caesar dressing

Whole grain wrap

Lasagna noodles

Ricotta cheese

Mozzarella cheese

Marinara sauce

Dark chocolate

Almonds

Feel free to adjust the meal plan and shopping lists according to your preferences and dietary needs.

CHAPTER TWELVE

Additional Tips for Success

Dining Out Strategies

Research Menus in Advance: Many restaurants post their menus online. Before you leave, look for healthier options.

Ask for Modifications: Don't hesitate to ask for substitutions, such as steamed vegetables instead of fries or dressing on the side.

Watch Portion Sizes: Restaurant portions can be large. Think about splitting a dish or bringing part of your dinner home.

Choose Wisely: Opt for grilled, baked, or steamed dishes instead of fried or sautéed ones.

Skip the Bread Basket: Avoid unnecessary calories by passing on the bread or chips offered before your meal.

Managing Cravings

Stay Busy: Take part in activities that will keep your body and mind busy.

Healthy Alternatives: Satisfy sweet cravings with fruit or dark chocolate, and salty cravings with nuts or seeds.

Hydrate: Sometimes thirst is mistaken for hunger. After sipping a glass of water, see whether the craving goes away in a short while.

Mindful Eating: Pay attention to your food, savoring each bite and eating slowly to recognize when you're full.

Staying Hydrated

Carry a Water Bottle: Keep a reusable water bottle with you to sip throughout the day.

Set Reminders: Set up apps or phone alerts to serve as a regular reminder to sip water.

Flavor Your Water: Add a splash of lemon, lime, or cucumber to make water more appealing.

Track Your Intake: Keep a log of how much water you drink to ensure you're meeting your hydration goals.

Support Groups

Join Online Communities: Websites and social media groups dedicated to healthy eating and fitness can provide support and motivation.

Find Local Groups: Look for local clubs or organizations focused on health and wellness.

Use Apps: Fitness and nutrition apps can help track progress, set goals, and connect with others.

Consult Professionals: Nutritionists, dietitians, and fitness trainers can offer personalized advice and support.

Conclusion

Final Thoughts

Embarking on a journey towards better kidney health through mindful eating and consistent hydration is a significant and commendable step. By following a well-balanced meal plan, staying informed, and making conscious choices, you are investing in your overall well-being and longevity. Remember, small changes can lead to substantial improvements in your health.

Encouragement and Motivation

Celebrate Small Wins: Every positive choice you make is a step in the right direction. No matter how tiny it may appear, acknowledge and celebrate your progress.

Stay Positive: Focus on the benefits you're gaining rather than the sacrifices you're making. Visualize the healthy, vibrant life you're working towards.

Be Patient: Changes in health take time. Be patient with yourself and understand that setbacks are a natural part of the journey.

Seek Support: Never be afraid to ask for help and assistance from friends, family, or support groups.

Next Steps in Your Kidney Health Journey

Regular Check-Ups: Schedule regular appointments with your healthcare provider to monitor your kidney function and overall health.

Stay Educated: Keep learning about kidney health and nutrition. Knowledge is a powerful tool in maintaining and improving your well-being.

Adopt Healthy Habits: Incorporate regular physical activity, adequate sleep, and stress management techniques into your routine.

Track Your Progress: Keep a journal of your meals, water intake, and how you feel. You can maintain your motivation and make the required corrections by keeping track of your progress.

Adjust as Needed: Be flexible and willing to adapt your meal plans and strategies as you learn more about what works best for your body.

Consult Professionals: Work with nutritionists, dietitians, and other healthcare professionals to tailor your approach to your specific needs and goals.

By taking these steps, you're not only enhancing your kidney health but also improving your overall quality of life. Stay committed, stay motivated, and remember that every positive choice brings you closer to your health goals. You have the power to make a lasting impact on your well-being, and your journey toward better health is a journey worth taking.

www.ingramcontent.com/pod-product-compliance
Lightning Source LLC
Chambersburg PA
CBHW071943210526
45479CB00002B/795